AF265238

HOW TO
STOP SMOKING
FOREVER

Kick-start your future
health and happiness right now!

HOW TO
STOP SMOKING
FOREVER

Kick-start your future
health and happiness right now!

by

Stephen Batt

2nd edition

First Publication, 2018

Palaceno House
Auckland
New Zealand

ISBN 978-0-473-52302-2 (Softcover)
ISBN 978-0-473-52303-9 (Epub)
ISBN 978-0-473-52304-6 (Kindle)
ISBN 978-0-473-52305-3 (PDF)
ISBN 978-0-473-52306-0 (iBook)

StephenBatt.com

HowToStopSmokingForever.com

Available from Amazon.com

Why I Wrote This Book

I used to be a smoker. I smoked about 20 cigarettes a day for almost 20 years. If I went out for a few drinks that'd climb to about 30 or 40. Sometimes I'd wake up coughing and I'd have a cigarette before getting out of bed. I didn't think I'd ever figure out how to stop smoking forever. But I did.

I stopped smoking 15 years before writing this book.

One day a friend asked me how I stopped. That started an in-depth conversation and a serious evaluation of the differences between all the times I'd tried to give up smoking, but failed, and the time I actually stopped smoking forever.

I know for certain that I'll never smoke again. And I knew it straight away the last time I gave up. I knew it because my thought process was different that time. It was the real thing.

Now I've developed that process into a technique that I believe will work for all adult smokers.

It worked for me. It can work for you too.

This book is not for teenagers. They know they're bulletproof and the future isn't really real. And it's not for people who don't really want to give up. It's for adults who genuinely want to quit.

Please read this book in its entirety, **from the beginning**, **NO SKIMMING**. If you do that I sincerely believe you will succeed.

At this point an author may wish you happy reading. But it's not that sort of book. There are no jokes. But it should lead to a very happy ending.

When you're smoke free I'd love to hear from you, because it makes me feel good to think I might have helped someone.

Either contact me through my website at

stephenbatt.com

or leave a review at Amazon.com

Or both.

THIS BOOK WAS WRITTEN FOR
ADULT SMOKERS WHO SERIOUSLY
WANT TO QUIT.

BE SURE TO READ IT IN THE ORDER
IT'S WRITTEN.

SKIMMING THROUGH OR READING
EXCERPTS WILL SERIOUSLY REDUCE
ITS EFFECTIVENESS.

Four Simple Steps
to
Stop Smoking
Forever

1. Read this book.

2. Read the Quitting Timetable and use the Progress Chart Instructions to personalize your Progress Chart.

3. Follow you personalized Progress Chart.

4. Stop Smoking Forever.

Contents

1. Statistics - Who Cares?

Most books about smoking are full of statistics.

People don't believe in statistics.

If we did we wouldn't buy lottery tickets.

But we do believe we might beat the odds. If we didn't think so, casinos and lotteries wouldn't be such big business.

So this book won't spend much time on statistics. There are however, just a couple of simple statistics that are worth bearing in mind.

Research shows that 1 in 2 adult smokers will die of smoking. Of those, half will die in middle age. That means that 1 in 4 smokers will lose about 30 years of life.

This book was written for adult smokers. Half of you will be killed by smoking if you don't give up. You know another adult smoker? Who's it going to kill, you or them?

Them obviously. You can beat the odds, right? Of course.

It couldn't happen to me.

Here's a little scenario for the gambler in all of us.

What if you got the opportunity to buy a ticket in a lottery where the first prize is $1,000,000. There's no second prize. The tickets are cheap. And there are only two of them. Would you buy a ticket?

Absolutely.

What if you got the chance to buy a ticket in the same lottery, with the $1,000,000 first prize, only two tickets, but the second "prize" was slowly dying over a period of about ten years, with ever increasing discomfort and pain?

Hmmmm. Maybe. All or nothing. Depends how desperate you're feeling.

What about if the second prize stayed the same, (slowly dying over a period of about ten years, with ever increasing discomfort and pain) but the first prize was frequent coughing, breathlessness, and general all round poor health. Would you buy a ticket in that lottery?

Well you do. Every time you buy a packet of cigarettes.

Not a problem. Odds are for beating. 1 in 2 smokers. You or them. Them, right?

So there's no point in dwelling here too long. Besides, if you didn't already think it's a good idea to give up smoking you wouldn't have opened the book.

So how do you stop?

Before we get to that point it makes sense to have a look at some of the more common methods that people use to try to give up. And to look at why they don't usually work.

2. How Not To Stop Forever

There are many familiar methods which people use time and time again in an effort to stop. These include:

Bets

Cutting down

Nicotine substitutes

I'll do it later

Let's all give up together

Bets

Bets usually have a time period attached, the implication being that after a certain time you'll get to have a cigarette again. Or if you can hold out just a little longer than the other person, you'll get the double reward - the money and a guilt-free cigarette.

Some thought patterns associated with bets:

"Well it's only fifty bucks. Who cares?"

or

"I'll win my bet at the end of March. That's this Friday. Phew. Not long to go. I can hold out till then. April 1st I can have a cigarette without it costing me anything." Really smart.

Cutting down

The theory behind cutting down (without a firm plan and a specific stopping date) is that when you become "less addicted" it will be much easier to give up from there. This leads to thinking that maybe you won't even have to give up at all. After all, if it's under control why stop? If you only smoke "socially" (yeah, really) then the occasional cigarette won't do much harm, right?

"Cutting down" is the opposite of "easing back up". There isn't even a term for that - smoking a few extras.

Except cutting down is harder. And pointless.

Cutting down without a specified end date doesn't work. Every smoker who has ever "cut down" has always "eased back up". When you try to cut down you are subconsciously telling yourself that you are not giving up, (which you're not), so you don't.

Nicotine substitutes

Here the idea is that the real problem is one of physical addiction to a substance. It doesn't address the psychological addiction which is far stronger in most people. Recovering heroin addicts don't automatically reach for a syringe each time they have a cup of tea or coffee. Or wonder what to do with their hands when chatting in a social environment.

Getting off cigarettes and onto patches is like a heroin addict giving up the needle but continuing to use heroin (maybe by smoking it).

I'll do it later ("When I'm past this stressful bit.")

Any excuse to delay the difficult is a good excuse. If you say you'll do it later it means that you don't have to address the problem at all right now. It's great. No guilt at all.

Trouble is when you get to feeling totally stress- free the first thing you feel like doing is relaxing with a cigarette. But even thinking about the consequences of smoking (which is a part of any real quitting decision) is pretty stressful in itself. Oh dear. Light up a stress reliever.

There's a lot of truth in proverbs - it's why they get repeated over the ages. "Never put off until tomorrow what you can do today." Why? Because you can't put off the damage being done by smoking until tomorrow.

If you decide to weed your garden next week, will the weeds stop growing for a week to wait for you? If you keep putting it off, how will it look in a year? Chances are that the weeds will have taken over and killed all your flowers. Still you can always rip everything out and plant a new garden. It's less traumatic than a lung transplant.

Lets all give up together

Some experts recommend this method. You can all keep a check on each other, encourage each other, console each other. But often it's two or three people who work together who try to quit together. Which is fine until they go out for a few drinks after work. Then it's - "Go on. You have one and I'll have one." And when another member of the group finds out they say - "Well to hell with you cheaters", and they have one too.

Who are you doing this for? What if you want to keep at it and the rest of the team decides to have a smoke. With a commitment to a team resolve rather than personal resolve, this group of people can decide for you that you're going to start smoking again.

There is one major reason why none of these methods really works:

You don't accept that the responsibility for <u>you</u> quitting is yours alone, and yours right now.

So that when one of these methods doesn't work you can blame some other person or circumstance.

Even if you don't say it. Subconsciously you believe it wasn't your fault.

By using any technique where you don't take personal responsibility for success or failure you don't have an inner belief and commitment.

And you won't give up smoking forever unless you have an inner belief and commitment that you have smoked your last cigarette.

Some of the above methods have worked occasionally for some people and that's good. But almost certainly these people had also reached a point of inner commitment to quitting. And then used one of these methods as a tool to help them implement it.

So how do you get this inner commitment and belief? How do you face up to taking the responsibility?

By taking a serious look at reality and choosing your future.

3. Facing reality – Choosing your future

You owe it to yourself to read this section right through at least once.

You will almost certainly find it distasteful, even horrible to the point of making you feel sick. It will be hard to read. It will be easier to put it down and not think about it. The tougher it is for you to read, the better. It means that you're taking it seriously enough already to make quitting that much easier.

By saying ooh, yuk, turning away and putting it out of your mind, it's very likely to come back to haunt you. Well worse than haunt you - kill you actually. Slowly and painfully.

And besides, if it's hard to read about, imagine what it's like to actually live (or rather die) through. Which is what you must do. Actually imagine what it's like. Immerse yourself in it.

The problem is if it doesn't upset you. That probably means that your head is buried in the sand. The "couldn't happen to me" syndrome.

Even if you don't think that you care about yourself, think about your family who'll have to nurse you and grieve and suffer and cry with you. You should at least consider what you may be going to put them through.

In any case it will certainly be better to feel temporarily sick while reading than to risk becoming actually, permanently sick by not reading about it. So get involved in this part.

Say to yourself -

"This is what will actually happen to me if I continue to smoke."

Cancer   Bronchitis   Heart Disease

Emphysema   Arterial Disease   Angina

Blah Blah Blah. So what. Big words. So you die. We've all got to die one day.

Which is perfectly true. But what that attitude ignores is how you die and when you die.

What is it actually like to die of one of the big words?

What is it actually like to become a smoking casualty?

Remember to take this section very personally. Don't sit back as an impartial observer. That attitude will not help you. To get the maximum benefit, try to imagine it's really happening to you. Immerse yourself in it completely. Remember it's not meant to be fun, or pleasant

The Smoker's Fitness Trail

You may be at any point along the trail. You may even just be at the very beginning of it. But it's a path you'll follow right to the end if you continue to smoke.

Hopefully you're not too far along it, because the point at which the damage becomes irreversible isn't a really long way from the start.

Regardless of how far along you are, it's just as important to stop. It doesn't ever get to be too late. Whenever you stop smoking, you stop doing damage, and your health will improve.

If you've already killed some lung tissue, the portion of lung that's already died will not recover, but if you continue to smoke, you'll kill even more.

Stage 1

After a few years of smoking, whenever you get a cold it goes to your chest.

Stage 2

Now when you get a cold, it's often a painfully uncomfortable chest infection. These last for two weeks, then four, then six as time goes by. They get harder to shake off. As well as deeper and more painful. Making it harder to smoke. But when they do clear up you go right back to smoking just as much as ever. That's if you didn't fight your way right through it by choking down a few ciggies to keep your body's nicotine balance organized. (Some smokers don't get sick very often at all. Lucky in the short term. But the path is the same later.)

Stage 3

After a while you never shake off that cough. It's there every morning. Your "Smoker's Cough". You'll adapt to this without too much trouble. A few good coughs and then the first ciggie of the day seems to get it back under control. Wasn't your body trying to tell you something? Like after eight hours of not having smoke forced through them, those poor suffering lungs would like to try to get rid of all the tar and mucus and bacteria that they'd rather not spend all day swimming in. Then you send in the gunboat, that first ciggie that quells the rioting for the day ahead. Followed up by regular patrols to keep the troublemakers in their place.

Stage 4

As the irritation caused by smoke to your lungs continues, you'll start to cough during the day as well. You'll be able to bring up sputum at any time of day. Isn't that great? Your lungs are still trying to tell you something, but you're not listening. The excess mucus that you are now producing provides food for bacteria. Infection is added to irritation. The mucus changes from clear to yellow. That's how you know that the bacteria are winning.

Stage 5

You'll start to suffer from respiratory infections that become more frequent, last longer and hurt more. The infection becomes deep enough to start destroying the lung walls. The longer you stay blocked up by mucus the greater and more permanent the damage becomes.

At this stage you will have already noticed how easily you become short of breath when walking up a hill or a flight of stairs. It'll make you cough.

You'll get tired more easily and start to avoid activities that involve any sort of exercise, even ones that you used to really enjoy. This will even get to include (or rather exclude) having sex - is that next ciggie really better than sex?

Stage 6

Even minor exertion or any sort of hurrying will produce more severe shortage of breath - you'll feel as though you are choking, like your air supply has been cut off.

So you've smoked yourself to a point where you can still look after yourself, provided there are no physical requirements placed on your body.

For the time being. How do you feel so far?

This is **your** life remember. **Your** future.

Stage 7

Eventually just breathing becomes slow and difficult and an unpleasant effort in itself.

Now it's official. You've got emphysema, or bronchitis, or possibly both. So you seek medical help. And if you think what you're reading now is bad enough, imagine how you'll feel when every doctor and nurse you see - and there'll be plenty of them - remind you that you've done this to yourself.

Stage 8

Now the whole focus of your life shifts to one thing. Life itself - staying alive. Whatever you used to do, whatever you were interested in, doesn't rate any more. Now you've got a full time job to keep breathing.

Put your hand over your mouth tightly. Block your nose. Breath only that air that you can force through your fingers. Do it for two minutes if you can.

How does it feel?

Welcome to your future.

You may have to feel like this, and getting progressively worse, twenty-four hours a day, for ten years before you eventually die.

How long you have to smoke to get to each stage on the path varies a lot, not only with what and how much you smoke, but with individuals who smoke the same amount. But that's not so important. What is important, is that by smoking, this is the path that you will travel. Smoking has this effect on your lungs.

This is not the lottery stage. This will happen to you if you continue to smoke - if you're lucky.

If you're not lucky - make that if you're not very lucky - you'll get cancer or heart disease or arterial disease. That's in addition to the above.

There's no point in spending too long on what will happen if you're not lucky, because we're all lucky. "It couldn't happen to me." "I might win lotto next week."

But if by some cruel twist of fate, you fall into that unlikely category of smokers who are killed by smoking (was it going to be you or that other smoker you know - remember the odds - 1 in 2) it will go something like this:

After ten or fifteen years of suffering (try to imagine what that'd be like), you'll die.

Suffering and pain are interesting concepts. It doesn't matter how hard you try, you can't imagine real pain. If you remember back to a serious injury in your past you can certainly remember that it wasn't any fun, but you really can't summon up an accurate mental picture of what that pain was like.

This doesn't mean that future pain and suffering won't be too bad. Or that old people don't mind pain so much.

If you die of emphysema or bronchitis you'll spend the last ten years of your life with only one daily objective - to keep breathing. It seems strange from this distance to think that you could struggle day in, day out, just to stay alive when you know that you'll never get better.

You are just prolonging death and there won't be any opportunities for any fun between now and the end. Forget going for a walk to the shop, a walk around the garden, or visiting your family, you'll just have to hope that they'll take pity and come and visit you, painful as that may be for them.

The fun's over. Forever. Yet people struggle on for years using all sorts of treatments and equipment - because they don't want to die.

You'll end up having to sleep sitting up so you don't drown in the fluid that your lungs are swimming in. No rest even in sleep.

Or if you get cancer things are even worse. In a cruel twist of fate many smokers who require surgery to remove parts of their mouth, tongue, throat or voice box in order to stay alive are told by their surgeon that they can't have the operation unless they give up smoking. (The die-hards, or die-easies, are still smoking even at this late stage.) Can you imagine that? - "I won't cut your throat out unless you stop smoking."

Even at that point it doesn't seem to be any easier to give up. Seems crazy, but some people even smoke through that hole in the front of their neck after they've had their voice box cut out.

It's not going to get any easier to give up than it is right now. That's the truth. It will never be any easier to give up than it is right now.

You may start getting sore legs or feet. As they get more painful, with attacks of pins and needles you'll find out that you have arterial disease. Then you'll start losing the feeling in your toes and feet as gangrene sets in. The only course of action at this point is amputation. Is that cigarette really worth losing your legs for?

Or, without any warning you get terrific pains in your chest. You start to perspire, to panic. It feels like you're having the life crushed out of you. Your chest is caving in. You feel like you are suffocating. You are overcome with an overwhelming feeling of fear and impending doom. A heart attack. Life will never be the same again.

Now that the consequences of smoking are so widely known, there is a growing tendency for doctors to refuse to commit large chunks of the public health budget (in those countries that have one) to keeping smokers alive.

And even when you get treatment it's not necessarily good news. There are a wide variety of treatments for all sorts of smoking induced illnesses but the one thing that they have in common is side effects. These are all different but include stomach pain, vomiting, confusion, irritability, fatigue, inability to sleep, shaking, headaches, muscle cramps, fever, itching, diarrhea, hearing loss, dizziness, hair loss, and disfigurement.

If you think it will help you to dwell more on this aspect of life and death, go to your local hospital and take a walk through the respiratory and surgical wards.

But more realistically because we don't really believe the worst case scenario will happen to us we'll just recap on the best case scenario.

That's the one where you cough more, walking up stairs becomes hard work, breathing itself gets difficult and you have to give up doing a lot of fun recreational pursuits like sport and sex.

Do you see yourself in ten years time as an invalid who can't have fun any more, or as someone that plays golf, or tennis, or whatever activity you enjoy, and has a good sex life? That's the choice you are faced with - today. The decision you are making right now.

If you don't face that choice, you'll be left with no choice. By continuing to smoke you are choosing a very unpleasant future.

So what are the alternative futures? Simple, really. A future involving fitness, health and vitality. We've all seen those wonderful healthy looking older people out walking in the park. Enjoying life. A future where you can do what you want to do. Unencumbered by disease.

Or the opposite.

You have two possible futures. The healthy future or the sick future. It's your choice. And now that you've spent a little bit of time having a serious look at what a sick future might be like, it's a choice that you have to make. You can't ignore it any more. Not - "I never thought about it really." It's too late for that. You've read about it now, you've thought about it and now it's up to you to choose. A sick future or a healthy future?

One of these futures WILL happen to you. And it is up to you which one. It is not fate or chance. It is <u>your choice</u>.

This is your life. Your one and only shot at it. If you destroy this body of yours, that's it. No second chances.

Get to grips with the reality. With almost anything else you get a second chance. House burns down - build another one. Lose your job - get another one. Lose all your money - start again.

But wreck your lungs, your throat, your heart, your legs, that's it. For ever. Gone. Damage done. You'll never ever ever be fully healthy again. You'll start to suffer and the suffering will end in death.

And the worst part is that if you wait until the symptoms appear, you've waited too long. The damage has started. The rot has set in. All you can do at that point is try to stop it getting worse.

If it's a little bit sudden for the reality of this to sink in you may need time to dwell on it. Don't finish the book yet. Read Section 3 again. You won't be ready for the next section until you've really got to grips with the reality of this one. Read it again tomorrow. And the next day. Until the reality sinks in. Read it every day for a month if necessary. And think about your options every time you have a cigarette. You just might find that they don't taste quite so good any more.

This is the most important choice you will make in your whole life. But you only have to make the right choice once. You can make the wrong choice thousands of times over. Every time you light a cigarette, you're making the wrong decision. 100% wrong. The worst decision you've ever made. And you're making that wrong decision over and over and over again.

Or you can make the right decision just once. It's the tough decision. But make the right choice and you only have to make it once.

Only when you have got to grips with the idea of the reality of your future and your control over it are you ready for Section 4.

Which is the easy bit. And you don't get to go to the easy bit until you've dealt with the hard bit.

So no cheating now. But when you're ready....

Just before we leave this bit, a few final thoughts.

What we're really dealing with here is your ability to control your life. So that you make it happen how you want it to happen. So that it's not something that happens to you.

It's your life. Take control. Be positive. Visualize your future as you want it to be. As you are going to make it.

Most people's goals are usually financial - "He who dies with the most toys wins" - measuring success with money.

But how successful is anybody who spends the last ten to fifteen years of their life suffering? Because it's not as if you suffer for a while and then you stop suffering and get up out of bed and go out and spend your millions and start having a great time again. You suffer and you suffer and you suffer and you die.

So who's the most successful? The contented old woman whiling away her twilight years gardening or playing bowls or sitting in the conservatory reading and reflecting on life through the wisdom of the years. Or the multi-millionaire, twenty years her junior who's had to give up doing all the things he loved doing most, just to concentrate his efforts on staying alive, hoping that his latest medication won't upset his pacemaker.

(In the real world most people who succeed financially understand that they are in control of their own destiny and don't smoke.)

Now we can move on to the more pleasant part of the book.

4. When to Stop

Just in case you're skimming -

DO NOT READ THIS SECTION UNLESS YOU'VE READ THE PREVIOUS SECTIONS FIRST.

This really is the easy bit provided you've got to grips with the realities of Section 3.

If you've decided on the sick future option, thank you for reading. There's nothing else in this book for you.

If you've decided on the healthy future option, you have come to the realization that you MUST stop smoking. Not that you'd LIKE TO give up. If that's where you're at, go back to section 3. When you KNOW that you are going to stop, there is only one decision left to make. When.

And that's not too difficult. When you know you've got to do something, especially if it's something that you'd rather not do, it's best to get it out of the way.

Get on with it. Do it. Start right now! Pick a day to start the program, preferably today. Tomorrow at the latest.

There's never going to be an easier time. You may think of excuses why there may be, but excuses only lead to a sick future, so why put it off? You know you've got to do it. The sooner it's behind you the better. Do it now.

If it seems too drastic, go back to Section 3. Read it every day. Get into it. Believe it. Don't say - "It couldn't happen to me." Say - "This is real. If I don't do something about it, it will happen to me." It's actually happening to millions of people around the world right now.

Keep this book by your bed. Or on your kitchen table. Take it to work. Read it every day.

Every time you pick up a cigarette, look at it first. Before you light it, ask yourself the question. What's my quality of life going to be like ten or twenty years from today? Healthy fun or sick misery.

Every cigarette is a decision.

Don't smoke another one without consciously making that decision.

Don't let the most important decision in your life be an unconscious one. Sick future or healthy future? Keep at it until it becomes real. Because it is real.

Then you'll stop.

And you may well find that it's not as hard as you thought it would be.

Many smokers who come to understand their two possible futures have found quite a surprising thing. When they understood that they weren't just trying to give up this time, that they were really giving up, that it was over, and they knew it for a fact, they felt quite different from all previous half-hearted attempts.

There were far less withdrawal symptoms than ever before.

In some cases, none at all.

No wild uncontrollable cravings.

Sure there'll be many times, especially in your early days as a non-smoker, when you really feel like having a cigarette. But it won't be too difficult to overcome. Because every time gets a little easier, and you know that the urge will go away.

For most people who give up smoking the first few days are the most difficult. The next couple of weeks can be quite difficult. And it gets progressively easier from there. Which is something to look forward to.

After a while it becomes easy, simple, not an issue at all. And you realize that not only will you never have another cigarette again, you won't even want to.

So when do you give up? As soon as you've got to grips with the reality of your future. Of your own mortality and human frailty.

Until you really deeply believe that you must give up and that you are going to stop forever, you're wasting your time trying. Each time you "try" to give up and fail, you reaffirm to yourself how difficult it is.

It's not. You've just got to be sure about what you're doing.

Don't try to do it. DO IT. Stop smoking for ever.

Don't ever smoke again. Not the odd one. Not - "I'll see how it goes for a couple of weeks." Not ever.

In this part the news keeps getting better.

Because once you stop - that means really stop, not just another attempt - you start feeling better immediately. So while those little cravings pop up from time to time to remind you that you'd like a cigarette, your general feeling of wellbeing reminds you that you'd rather not actually smoke it. The fantastic feeling of health and fitness is something a smoker can't buy for a million bucks.

And you get a wonderful feeling of achievement.

Which is great for your self esteem. "Hey, if I can do this (which is generally accepted as being hugely difficult and something that many people try and fail) by really applying my mind to it, what else can I achieve if I really put my mind to it?"

What if you buckle and have a cigarette?

The hardest time for most people "trying" to give up smoking is the first time they go out and have a couple of drinks. Not only is the desire at its greatest but the will is at its weakest. Many fold and smoke one or two or ten. And the next day give it no more thought than "I tried and failed." And so they start smoking again.

Wrong.

You're much further ahead than you were when you gave up in the first place. It's much easier to do it from here than if you get back into it.

So pick up the book again. Reaffirm your belief in reality. And look on your moment of weakness as a minor glitch. Not as confirmation that you are a real deep down fundamental smoker. There is no such thing. We weren't designed to smoke. None of us. That's why it makes us cough. And makes us sick. And ultimately kills us.

So keep this book handy for emergencies. Any time you feel yourself weakening, read it again. Read it instead of smoking the cigarette mounted in the glass case - better still, if you've got one of those, take the cigarette out and put the book in.

Hopefully you'll never need to look at it again. Because you will know, deep inside, that you'll never smoke again.

5. How to Stop

Once again - just in case you're skimming -

DO NOT READ THIS SECTION UNLESS YOU'VE READ THE PREVIOUS SECTIONS FIRST.

If you've gone straight to here looking for the quick answer, you're only kidding yourself.

It doesn't work that way. If it did, this would be the only section in the book.

Once you realize that you have two possible futures and that the responsibility for your chosen future is yours and yours alone you are ready...

Follow These Steps

to

Stop Smoking

Forever

1. Provided you've read the book and decided that you MUST STOP smoking, then...

2. Read the Quitting Timetable and use the Progress Chart Instructions to personalize your Progress Chart.

3. Follow your personalized Progress Chart. Smoke no more than the number of cigarettes you have allowed for yourself.

4. Stop Smoking Forever.

The Quitting Timetable

To allow your mind and body to get used to the new sensation of not smoking, it helps to take a graduated approach.

Day 1 - Cut down to half the amount you normally smoke. Be honest - if you're not, you're only fooling yourself.

Days 2-6 Continue to smoke no more than half your regular amount.

Day 7 - Cut the number smoked in half again.

Day 14 - Cut the number smoked in half again.

Day 18 - Cut the number smoked in half again.

Day 21 - Cut the number smoked in half again.

Day 28 - Stop smoking forever.

Any time you feel a strong urge to smoke, remind yourself why you don't smoke any more, by re-reading the book.

Progress Chart Instructions

1. Now that you've decided that you're going to stop smoking forever, use a calendar to choose a day and date to start the program, preferably within the next 2 days.

2. Print a copy of the blank Progress Chart on page 53.

For A4 or US letter size print at 160%.

3. Write your chosen starting day in the Weekday column next to Day 1. (Refer to Example Progress Chart)

4. Fill in the remainder of the Weekday column.

5. Write your chosen starting date in the Date column next to your starting day.

6.   Fill in the remainder of the Date column and the Month column.

7. Fill in the Cigarette Allowance column.

How many cigarettes do you usually smoke in a day? Write half this number in the spaces corresponding to days 1 through 6. Halve the number again and write it in the spaces corresponding to days 7 through 13. Once again, halve the number and write it in the spaces corresponding to days 14 through 20. Once again, halve the number and write it in the spaces corresponding to days 21 through 27.

9. Your Progress Chart is now ready.

Put it up on your fridge door or somewhere that you'll see it often.

Smoke no more than the number of cigarettes in the Cigarette Allowance column.

Monitor your progress by counting how many cigarettes you actually smoke during the course of the day and fill in the Cigarettes Smoked column as you go.

You may be able to beat your allowance. If so, great.

Go for it! Go for a healthy future.

Thanks for reading.

REVIEWS are the best way to help others find the sort of books they may be looking for.

A review that's brief, just a sentence or two, will let other readers know what you liked about the book, and why they might like it too.

So if you think this book's worth reading, please leave a review (or at least a rating) at Amazon.com or Goodreads.com or anywhere else that you can.

And PLEASE DO IT RIGHT NOW before you forget (you know you will).

Thanks again

Stephen Batt

Progress Chart

Day	Weekday	Date	Month	Cigarette Allowance	Cigarettes Smoked	Day
1						1
2						2
3						3
4						4
5						5
6						6
7						7
8						8
9						9
10						10
11						11
12						12
13						13
14						14
15						15
16						16
17						17
18						18
19						19
20						20
21						21
22						22
23						23
24						24
25						25
26						26
27						27
28						28
				0		

Progress Chart Example

For a 40 cigarette per day smoker

Day	Weekday	Date	Month	Cigarette Allowance	Cigarettes Smoked	Day
1	Wednesday	18	September	20		1
2	Thursday	19		20		2
3	Friday	20		20		3
4	Saturday	21		20		4
5	Sunday	22		20		5
6	Monday	23		20		6
7	Tuesday	24		10		7
8	Wednesday	25		10		8
9	Thursday	26		10		9
10	Friday	27		10		10
11	Saturday	28		10		11
12	Sunday	29		10		12
13	Monday	30		10		13
14	Tuesday	1	October	5		14
15	Wednesday	2		5		15
16	Thursday	3		5		16
17	Friday	4		5		17
18	Saturday	5		5		18
19	Sunday	6		5		19
20	Monday	7		5		20
21	Tuesday	8		2		21
22	Wednesday	9		2		22
23	Thursday	10		2		23
24	Friday	11		2		24
25	Saturday	12		2		25
26	Sunday	13		2		26
27	Monday	14		2		27
28	Tuesday	15		1		28
				0